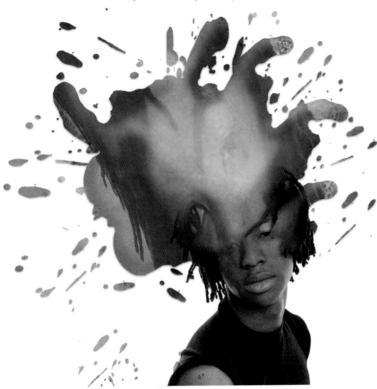

Incredibly Disgusting Drugs™

Speed

Edward Willett

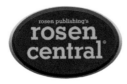

rosen publishing's
rosen central®

New York

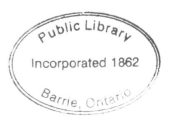

Published in 2008 by The Rosen Publishing Group, Inc.
29 East 21st Street, New York, NY 10010

Copyright © 2008 by The Rosen Publishing Group, Inc.

First Edition

Library of Congress Cataloging-in-Publication Data

Willett, Edward.
Speed / Edward Willett. — 1st ed.
    p. cm. — (Incredibly disgusting drugs)
Includes bibliographical references and index.
ISBN-13: 978-1-4042-1377-7 (library binding)
1. Methamphetamine—United States. 2. Methamphetamine abuse—United States.
I. Title.
HV5822.A5W55 2008
616.86'40973—dc22

                                                              2007035112

Manufactured in the United States of America

Contents

Introduction

peed. Meth. Chalk. Ice. Crystal. Crank. Glass. These are just some of the many names for the closely related drugs known technically as amphetamines and methamphetamines. However, they all add up to the same result: bad news.

Amphetamines have been around since the late nineteenth century. They have been abused for almost as long as the drug has existed. Amphetamines were originally used to treat bronchial and nasal congestion in the 1930s. It didn't take users much time to find out that the drug also increased alertness, decreased appetite, and in general made them feel good. In the last few decades, methamphetamine, an even more potent stimulant, has become the form of speed most often abused.

There's no question that speed makes people feel good—but only for a short time and only at a terrible cost. Soon, users need more and more of it to get the same effect. They begin to crave it to the point where they will neglect their jobs, their families, and even their own bodies. Some meth users' teeth actually rot and fall out of their mouths. The users are too focused on getting speed to remember to brush or floss. The drug can also make them crave sugary foods and drinks.

Speed rewires the brain, interfering with its usual operation. Some of the changes may be permanent. The bad effects include memory loss, aggression, and psychotic behavior. Because speed stimulates the whole body, it can lead to heart damage. It suppresses appetite, which can produce malnutrition. And an overdose of speed can kill.

Users will cheat and steal to support their habit. They're also more likely to be involved in violence because the drug makes them aggressive. Methamphetamine is often cooked up in home laboratories that produce not only speed (which is bad enough), but also toxic fumes and liquid waste that can poison an entire house and the environment.

Wherever speed abuse goes, crime, unemployment, child neglect or abuse, and other ills follow. Speed addiction can be treated, but it's not easy. It's much better not to touch the drug in the first place. And the more you know about it, the more likely it is you'll steer clear. This book will teach you about speed: what it is, what it does, and just how disgusting it really is.

1

What Is
Speed?

Speed is one of the street names for two related classes of man-made drugs: amphetamines and methamphetamines. Amphetamine was first synthesized, or manufactured, at the University of Berlin in Germany by chemist Lazar Edeleanu in 1887. His name for the compound was phenylisopropylamine.

Just two years previously, noted Japanese chemist Nagayoshi Nagai had purified ephedrine from a shrub native to South Asia called *Ephedra distachya*. Ephedrine is the active substance in various traditional medicines in the region. It's a stimulant, which means it promotes wakefulness and alertness.

Methamphetamine is closely related to amphetamine. Nagai synthesized methamphetamine for the first time in 1893. Another Japanese chemist, Akira Ogata, synthesized a more potent, crystallized form of methamphetamine—now known as crystal meth—in 1919.

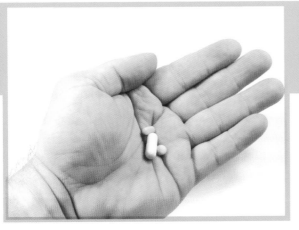

For many years, amphetamines were available over the counter as stimulants and diet pills.

No use was found for amphetamines in Western medicine until 1928. That year, the pharmaceutical company Smith, Kline, and French introduced Benzedrine. Sold in inhalers over the counter (without a doctor's prescription), it was used to treat nasal and bronchial congestion.

Benzedrine users soon discovered that the drug did more than just open up their breathing passages. It also acted as a stimulant, making them more active and talkative. It decreased appetite and, in general, just made them feel good.

The First Abuse: Bennies

Because of its effect as a stimulant and widespread use in inhalers, Benzedrine became the first form of amphetamine to be abused. People would crack open the inhalers and remove the Benzedrine-soaked paper strips inside. Then they'd roll the strips into small balls and swallow them like pills, either by themselves or with coffee and alcohol. The drug got the nickname "Bennies." You may run across the term in books and movies set in the mid-twentieth century.

The stimulant effects that led people to abuse amphetamine also made it useful in treating narcolepsy. (Narcolepsy is a brain-related condition that causes people to suddenly drop off to sleep at inappropriate times.) Benzedrine's manufacturer began making the drug in pill form. Some doctors also prescribed Benzedrine as a diet pill to suppress the appetite.

During the Second World War (1939–1945), many countries' militaries provided amphetamine and methamphetamine to their troops as stimulants. In the German military, for instance, chocolates dosed with methamphetamine were given to pilots and tank crews, among others, to help keep them awake during battles. German chancellor Adolf Hitler took methamphetamine daily from 1942 until his death in 1945.

Partly because of their military use, amphetamine and methamphetamine, which earned the nickname "speed," were widely available in the years after the war. Both drugs were legal then. (Some universities reportedly even handed out speed at exam time to help students stay awake for studying.)

In the late 1950s and early 1960s, speed became the drug of choice of the countercultural Beat movement, whose followers were called "beatniks" by the mainstream press.

As reports began to emerge in the 1940s and 1950s about rising Benzedrine abuse, doctors stopped suggesting it as relief for nasal and bronchial congestion. In 1959, the U.S. Food and Drug Administration (FDA) banned purchase of the drug without a doctor's prescription.

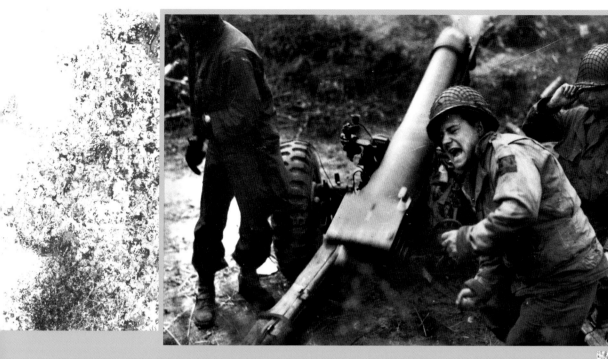

During the Second World War, many countries provided amphetamine and methamphetamine to their troops to help them stay alert during combat.

The Need for Regulation

In the 1960s, people began setting up secret, illegal laboratories so that they could make their own speed. In 1970, the U.S. Congress enacted the Comprehensive Drug Abuse Prevention and Control Act to help combat the abuse of drugs. (One part of this act, called Title II, is commonly known as the Controlled Substances Act.) This law regulated the manufacture, importation, possession, and distribution of certain substances and drugs,

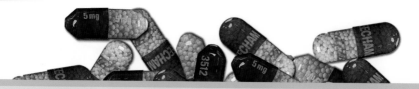

Speed in the Postwar Years

Even after amphetamines became prescription-only, they were frequently available and widely used. In 1967, about thirty-one million prescriptions were written for amphetamines in the form of diet pills. By 1969, more than 13 percent of American college students reported having used amphetamines at least once.

including amphetamine and methamphetamine. The law also required that every drug on the market be evaluated and placed into one of five categories based on how the drug was to be used, its safety issues, and its possibility for being addictive. Drugs in the first category, Schedule I, are thought to carry the highest risk to people, and those in Schedule V, the lowest.

Despite the enactment of the Comprehensive Drug Abuse Prevention and Control Act, the federal government found that it needed to make stricter laws to try to prevent further abuse. In 1996, the Comprehensive Methamphetamine Control Act became law, making it illegal to possess chemicals and equipment that could be used to make methamphetamine.

Ephedrine and pseudoephedrine, ingredients found in cold remedies such as Sudafed and Contac, have also been increasingly restricted because they can be used as the raw materials for making methamphetamine. Individuals can purchase only a limited amount of ephedrine- or pseudoephedrine-containing drugs within a specified time period. Drugstores have to store them securely to prevent their theft.

Today, amphetamine and methamphetamine have limited medical uses. They're sometimes prescribed for the treatment of attention-deficit/hyperactivity disorder (ADHD) and narcolepsy. They're sometimes used to supplement other treatments for depression. The FDA has listed them as Schedule II drugs and classified them as central nervous system (CNS) stimulants. Schedule II drugs are those that have a currently accepted medical use, but also have a high potential for abuse and a high likelihood of addiction.

2
Speed
and the Body

Speed affects the body in many different and nasty ways. All of those effects begin invisibly because they start inside the brain. To understand them, you have to know a little bit about how the brain works.

Neurons, Axons, and Dendrites

The brain is made up of billions of nerve cells, called neurons. Neurons have three main parts. The cell body contains the nucleus. Short fibers called dendrites receive messages from other neurons and pass them along to the cell body. The axon, a long fiber, carries messages from the cell body of one neuron to the dendrites of other neurons.

The axon of one neuron doesn't actually touch the dendrites of another. Instead, they are separated by a small space called a synapse. Messages are passed from an axon to another neuron's dendrites by chemicals

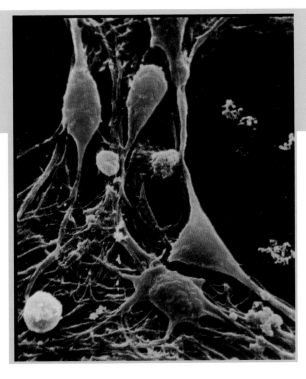

This scanning electron micrograph of nerve cells shows the large cell body, where the nucleus is located; the long, thick axons; and the smaller, branching dendrites.

called neurotransmitters. The neurotransmitter is released by the axon, crosses the synapse, and attaches to the dendrite at a specific place called a receptor. There are different receptors for different neuro-transmitters. Once the neurotransmitter has passed along its message by plugging into a receptor, it is either destroyed or returned to its originating neuron for reuse.

Dopamine

One neurotransmitter is called dopamine. Dopamine makes you feel good. If you score a goal in a hockey game, eat something you love, or share a laugh with a friend, some of the axons in your brain release dopamine to pass along this feeling of pleasure to other neurons. Then the dopamine is returned to the originating axon.

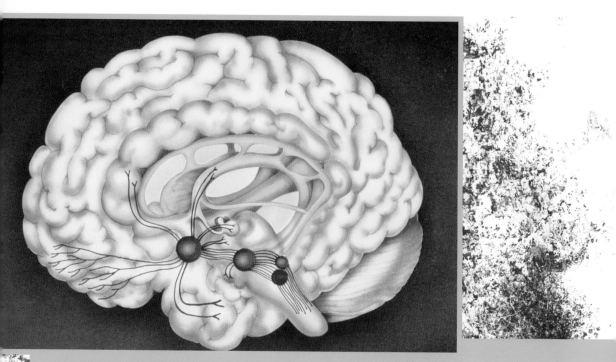

Different drugs affect different parts of the brain. For example, this diagram shows the regions of the brain, marked by red spheres, where painkilling drugs such as morphine take effect.

But when speed molecules make it into the brain, they disrupt this process. Amphetamines and methamphetamines have molecules that are very similar in shape, size, and chemical structure to those of dopamine. They are able to slip into the storage area for dopamine in axons, displacing the dopamine molecules and releasing them to surrounding dendrites. That causes more neurons to release dopamine, which triggers still more neurons to release dopamine, producing a domino effect. In other words, speed makes users feel a rush of pleasure, even though they haven't really done anything pleasurable.

The effect of dopamine is normally short-lived. Speed, however, remains active in the body for a long time. The effects of even a small dose can be felt for four to six hours. One reason for this is that the speed molecules also prevent the dopamine from being returned to the neurons for recycling. Furthermore, speed inhibits the action of an enzyme that helps break down the dopamine, which means it can remain active longer.

Because they cannot return to the neurons for recycling, however, the dopamine molecules are eventually destroyed. Because neurons normally recycle dopamine, it takes them a long time to rebuild their supply. This is why speed's feeling of euphoria—a feeling of elation or well-being—is followed by a "crash," a let-down feeling.

Noradrenaline

Speed's structure is also similar to another neurotransmitter, called noradrenaline. Noradrenaline is produced not only in the nerve cells in the brain, but also in the nerve cells throughout the body. (Dopamine is produced only by brain neurons.)

Because speed increases the release of, and effect of, noradrenaline throughout the body, it affects many body organs. Among the most significant effects are on the heart, which beats faster and starts contracting harder. This effect on the heart raises blood pressure. Noradrenaline also causes blood vessels to contract, which boosts

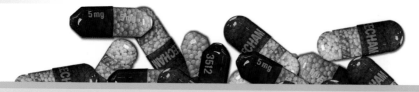

It Feels Like Adrenaline

Some of these effects are similar to those of adrenaline, the hormone that makes your heart pound when you're excited or scared. Adrenaline is part of the "fight-or-flight" mechanism that prepares you either to face danger or to run away from it. Adrenaline gives you a burst of energy just when you need it.

Speed mimics the effects of adrenaline because speed molecules are similar in structure to adrenaline molecules. The body can't tell the difference.

blood pressure even more. This combination can cause irregular heartbeats, chest pain, and even a heart attack.

Other effects of using speed can include dizziness, blurred vision, anxiety, restlessness, decreased appetite, difficulty sleeping, and tremors. Speed also raises the body temperature. Sometimes a user's fever soars so high, he or she goes into a convulsion, which is an uncontrollable shaking. Occasionally those convulsions are fatal.

Then, when the crash comes and the physical effects subside, users feel extremely fatigued. They often fall into a long but unrestful sleep. When they wake up, they may feel irritable and depressed. That combination may make the urge very strong to take speed again and rekindle the rush. Moreover, these physical effects of taking the drug are just those felt in the short term.

Long-Term Effects

Over the long term, the physical effects on the body and brain can become truly disgusting. Long-term use can permanently change the brain by damaging the neuron cell endings. The result can be difficulty understanding words and slower muscle movements. Long-term use can also result in inflammation of the heart lining and decreased sexual ability.

Users aren't putting just themselves at risk. Babies born to speed users are more likely to be premature and have a low birth weight, and they may be at increased risk of birth defects. They can even be born addicted to speed themselves and experience withdrawal symptoms, such as agitation and drowsiness. Speed-using mothers who nurse their babies continue to pass the drug on to them through their breast milk.

Over time, the abuse of speed can permanently damage a person's brain.

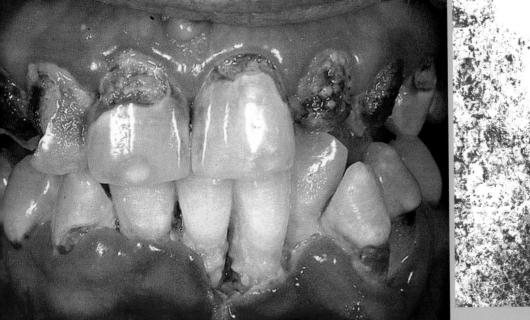

Meth mouth–rotting teeth and diseased gums–is one of the most disgusting effects of long-term speed abuse. A user can go from having healthy teeth to a mouth like the one shown in the photo above in a single year.

Meth Mouth

One of the ugliest effects of long-term speed abuse is severe dental problems, collectively known as meth mouth. According to the American Dental Association (ADA), methamphetamine users can go from having healthy teeth to having very sensitive teeth to losing teeth in about a year. Gum disease is also a common side effect of abusing speed.

Dr. Robert M. Brandjord, ADA president, put it this way: "Meth mouth robs people, especially young people, of their teeth and frequently leads to full-mouth extractions and a lifetime of wearing dentures."

Just how disgusting is meth mouth? Dr. Brandjord described it as "rampant tooth decay" and said meth users' teeth can end up "blackened, stained, rotting, crumbling, or falling apart."

There are several reasons for these harmful dental problems. For one, speed dries out a user's mouth. It also seems to cause a craving for high-calorie, carbonated beverages. It may also lead to tooth-grinding and clenching. Finally, speed users simply neglect toothbrushing and flossing for long periods of time. That's because they're more interested in getting their next dose of speed than they are in looking after their mouths—or any other part of their rapidly deteriorating bodies.

3
Effects
on the Mind

peed not only impacts the body, of course. It affects the mind, too, not just by producing a feeling of euphoria, but by changing users' personalities and how they relate to the world (and other people) around them.

Regular users of speed develop tolerance. That means they need to take the drug more frequently and/or take more of it each time to achieve the same sensation. After a while, users become dependent on speed. Their craving can become so intense, they'll go to great lengths to get more. They may cheat or steal from their friends, or commit crimes, to obtain money to buy the drug. At that point, they are said to be addicted.

The Rewired Brain of the User

Speed users are literally rewiring their brains. By scanning the brain activity of users, scientists have discovered that the drug changes the normal activity of the dopamine

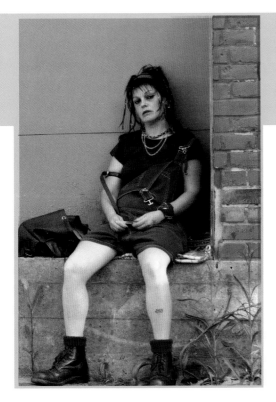

Long-term speed users lose interest in themselves, other people, and the world around them. All they can think about is finding their next dose of the drug.

system to the point that motor speed and verbal learning are both reduced.

Moreover, studies have revealed that chronic speed users suffer severe changes to the parts of the brain associated with emotion and memory. These changes probably account for many of the symptoms exhibited by chronic users. Those symptoms include memory loss and mood disturbances, such as irritability and nervousness. (Users may become so nervous that they physically twitch or shake.) Users may be easily distracted and have trouble focusing and remembering. Many users have trouble sleeping. Others alternate long periods of sleeplessness with long periods of sleep. Some users talk constantly.

Over time, heavy users can slip into various forms of psychosis, including paranoia (the irrational feeling that other people are trying to harm you), hallucinations, and repetitive motor activity (doing the same

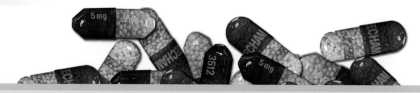

What Is an Addiction?

Addiction is a chronic, relapsing disease that causes people to engage in activities or consume substances harmful to their health and well-being. The word "chronic" means long-lasting and on-going, and the word "relapsing" means that people who suffer from addiction are always at risk of falling back into their bad habit.

There are many addictive drugs. Some cause only a psychological craving. Others, such as speed, actually change the user's body and brain, creating a physical need for the substance.

thing over and over again without being able to stop). Examples include picking at your skin, pulling out your hair, compulsively cleaning or grooming, or taking objects apart and putting them back together again. The paranoia and hallucinations can lead speed users to bizarre and sometimes violent behavior.

Good-bye to Family and Friends

All of these personality changes can drive away friends and family. That's all right with heavy speed users because for them, the drug is more important than personal relationships. It can also become more

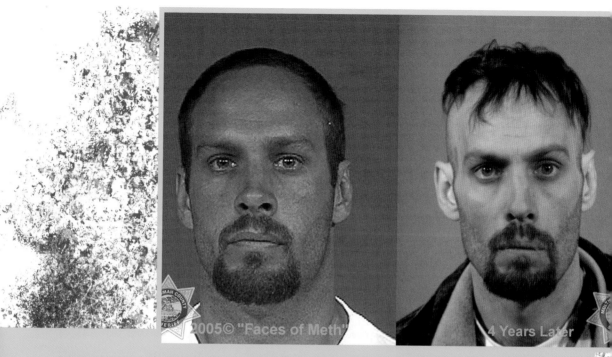

2005© "Faces of Meth"   4 Years Later

After four years of methamphetamine abuse, this man's appearance changed drastically because he paid little attention to his health and hygiene.

important than personal hygiene, eating, and safety. Users may become dirty, greasy-haired, and thin to the point of starvation. (And don't forget about meth mouth.)

Risk-taking behavior can lead to crippling or fatal accidents. The illusion of power and control that the drug provides can also lead users to engage in unsafe sex. That increases their risk of contracting sexually transmitted diseases, including AIDS.

Not surprisingly, speed users often have trouble doing their schoolwork or holding down a job.

Two Case Studies

Hayley and Lisa are two former speed users who described their experiences in *Drugs & Addiction Magazine*.

The first time she tried crystal meth, Hayley said, "It was wildly exciting. I felt free and untroubled. I felt like a different person when I was using—confident, sexy, and full of energy." But matters went downhill quickly. "My love of meth took me to the streets of downtown Vancouver [British Columbia] because that's where all the action was . . . The fighting, stealing, and sexual assaults came along as part of the package, but by then I was already sucked into that scene. At the time, my parents were going through a divorce, and I couldn't handle them anymore. So I left. The street was my new home."

Lisa was only in eighth grade when she saw her older sister and her sister's boyfriend smoking crystal meth. "Grade eight was my worst year. I was having a really hard time. I saw them and they looked happy . . . I figured I had nothing to lose. As soon as I could get it every day, I was a full-fledged addict."

But over time, Lisa said, "the highs were becoming shorter and shorter, and the lows were unbearable. I was anxious, depressed, and angry all the time, and the only thing that could bring me out of it was more drugs." She went to a former teacher and sought help.

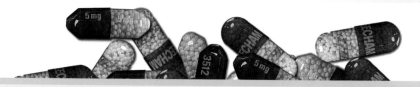

A Particularly Nasty Delusion

One of the nastiest delusions heavy speed abusers are subject to is formication. That's the scientific name for the feeling that insects are crawling all over your skin, even though there's nothing there. Speed users sometimes pick at these nonexistent insects so much that they break open their skin, forming scabs and scars.

Hayley stopped using for another reason: "I got caught stealing and I spent five nights in the youth jail. That was the worst experience of my life." When she got out, she was put into mandatory treatment.

Lisa's and Hayley's stories are far from unique. Speed in all its forms is among the most commonly abused drugs in North America.

4
Abusing
Speed

peed is widely abused. In fact, in many western and midwestern states, methamphetamine is the third-most abused drug after alcohol and marijuana.

Speed comes in many forms. Amphetamines are usually tablets or capsules. They may be prescription drugs, or they may be look-alike drugs cooked up in illegal labs.

Methamphetamine is almost always homemade and looks like a coarse powder, crystal, or chunks. It ranges in color from off-white to yellow, and it can be swallowed, snorted, or injected. The most potent form of methamphetamine is crystal meth, which is often used by addicts as a replacement for cocaine or is mixed with heroin. Its effects last longer than those of cocaine. It is sold as a powder that can be injected, inhaled, or swallowed. Finally, the most concentrated form of crystal meth is called "ice" or "glass" because

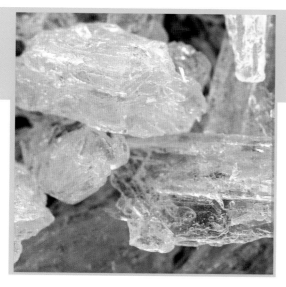

The most concentrated form of crystal meth is called "ice" or "glass" because that's what it looks like.

it resembles tiny chunks of translucent glass. It can be smoked rather than injected.

Smoking or injecting meth leads to a very fast uptake of the drug by the brain and produces a short-lived, but very intense, "rush" or "flash." Snorting or swallowing it produces a high, but not an intense rush. Snorting produces effects within three to five minutes. Swallowing produces effects within fifteen to twenty minutes.

How Many Users?

According to the 2004 National Survey on Drug Use and Health, approximately 11.7 million Americans ages twelve and older have tried methamphetamine at least once. That's 4.9 percent of the twelve-or-older population. What's more, approximately 1.4 million (0.6 percent of the twelve-or-older population) had used methamphetamine within the last year, and 583,000 (0.2 percent) within the past month.

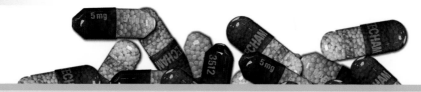

Speeding to the Emergency Room

According to the Drug Abuse Warning Network (DAWN), which collects information on drug-related episodes from hospital emergency departments throughout the United States, the number of emergency room visits related to speed abuse increased 50 percent between 1995 and 2002, reaching approximately 73,000. That's equivalent to 4 percent of all drug-related visits.

The number of people admitted to treatment programs for abusing speed has also increased. In 1992, approximately 21,000 speed users were admitted to treatment programs. That number represented a bit more than 1 percent of all treatment admissions that year. By 2004, the number had soared to 150,000 and represented 8 percent of all treatment admissions.

Canadian figures are similar. The 2004 Canadian Addiction Survey found that 6.4 percent of the Canadian population ages fifteen or older had used speed at least once.

That usage starts early. A 2005 study found that 3.1 percent of U.S. eighth graders, 4.1 percent of tenth graders, and 4.5 percent of twelfth graders had tried methamphetamine. High school students surveyed by the Centers for Disease Control and Prevention (CDC) that same year got

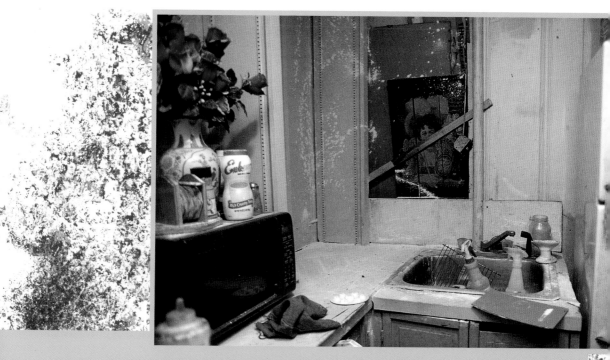

Debris litters the kitchen of a meth dealer and user. A lot of crystal meth is concocted in dangerous amateur laboratories like this one.

similar numbers: 6.2 percent reported using methamphetamine at some point. Nevertheless, on the plus side, that was down from 7.6 percent in 2003 and 9.8 percent in 2001.

Speed abuse continues to spread. The National Institute on Drug Abuse's Community Epidemiology Work Group, which tracks the nature and patterns of drug abuse in twenty-one major areas of the United States, reported in January 2006 that speed abuse is a particular problem in the West and continues to spread to other areas, rural and urban alike, in the South and Midwest. Methamphetamine abuse was reported to be the fastest-growing problem in metropolitan Atlanta, Georgia.

Who Uses Speed?

The average user of speed is a white person, in his or her twenties or thirties, who has a high school education or better, and who has a full- or part-time job. Almost as many women as men use speed: about 55 percent are male, and 45 percent are female.

Speed use is much more prevalent among people living on the street. A study in Vancouver, British Columbia, found that 72 percent of what they called "street-involved youth" (ages fourteen to thirty) used speed. A Toronto, Ontario, study found that 37 percent of seventy-six homeless young people surveyed used methamphetamine at least once each month.

Speed has a terrible effect on the people who use it. But speed also has a horrifying effect on the people who don't use it.

Meth Labs Are Poison

Methamphetamine is often made in illegal laboratories that can operate unnoticed within an otherwise ordinary neighborhood. The labs are environmental hazards. For every pound of meth produced, five to six pounds (almost three kilograms) of hazardous waste are generated. That's because the chemicals used to make meth are poisonous. These chemicals can include red phosphorous, hydrochloric acid, anhydrous ammonia, drain cleaner, battery acid, lye, lantern fuel, and antifreeze. Because the labs

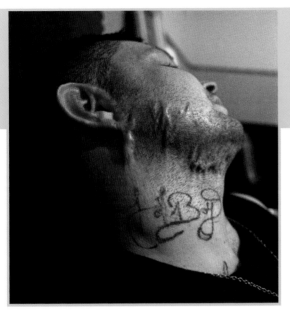

This long-term meth user is still horribly scarred from the burns he suffered over more than 40 percent of his body when the meth lab he was operating blew up.

are illegal, the people running them secretly dump the waste into streams, ponds, the sewage system, or on other people's property.

The labs also produce poisonous vapors that can seep into insulation and carpets, rendering whole buildings uninhabitable. It costs thousands of dollars and takes specialized training and equipment to clean up after a meth lab. Furthermore, property owners are often held liable for the cost of the cleanup. That means that a landlord whose tenants have been operating an illegal meth lab may face bills so high that he or she may lose the property altogether, or even go bankrupt.

Meth labs are also fire hazards and can possibly explode. Often, children are living in homes where meth labs operate. They frequently suffer from neglect because their family members or caregivers are more focused on using or making speed than looking after them. They are also at risk of being poisoned by the toxic fumes (which can cause brain damage),

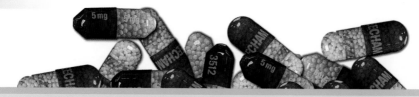

Speed May Speed AIDS

Speed abuse may actually worsen the progression of HIV, the virus that causes AIDS. In animal studies, methamphetamine made the virus multiply faster. Human speed users with HIV suffer more brain damage from the virus than nonusers.

overdosing on speed left lying around the house, or being killed or injured in a fire or explosion.

Many children whose parents make or use meth end up in foster homes. This circumstance puts a strain on the social services of their community. Such children often need special care: they may be malnourished and may have been physically or sexually abused. According to the *New York Times*, it can even be difficult to find foster parents for these children because of behavioral problems. They may have trouble sleeping in a bed because they're used to sleeping on the floor. They may not even have been toilet-trained.

Speed Leads to Crime

Speed users and makers contribute to crime within a community. Addicts may steal from their friends or family to pay for their habit, or resort to burglary or shoplifting. Speed users are often violent, posing a risk to

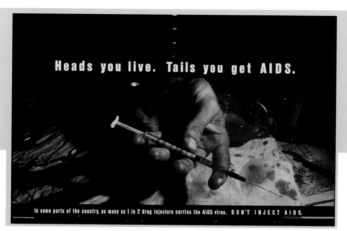

Heads you live. Tails you get AIDS.

In some parts of the country, as many as 1 in 2 drug injectors carries the AIDS virus. DON'T INJECT AIDS.

This poster warns of drug use and AIDS. Because users who inject speed often share needles, speed use contributes to the spread of AIDS.

other citizens and the police. Identity theft, domestic violence, and even murder can time and again be linked to speed use, trafficking, or manufacturing.

The health effects of speed use and the dangers of its manufacture also put a strain on the health-care services of communities. Speed use lowers inhibition, leading users to engage in dangerous behaviors, including unsafe sexual practices that contribute to the spread of sexually transmitted diseases such as hepatitis and AIDS. Users that inject the drug often share needles, which is another way to spread disease.

A Typical Tale of Speed Abuse

Eric Stone, now in his twenties, is a typical speed addict. He first tried meth in high school (along with many other drugs). He grew up in a small town. "I liked the way drugs made me think, feel, and behave," Stone wrote in a personal account posted on the Web site of the Partnership for a

Drug-Free America. "They gave me a false sense of security. No matter what was going wrong in my life, when I got high, it all went away."

But, he went on to say, it wasn't long after he started using that he discovered he could no longer get high the way he used to. Instead, he got paranoid, scared, and uncomfortable. Arrested several times, both for drug possession and stealing, Stone went in and out of juvenile detention centers and rehab clinics. Despite all that, he said, he still thought the answers to his problems lay in drugs.

"By 18," Stone said, "I was spiritually dead. I had experienced many bad highs and bad trips, dropped out of high school, lost my popularity and friends, and spent most of my time isolating myself in my room using more drugs."

He stole from his mother and lied to her to the point where she filed a restraining order and had the police force him out of her home. After Stone dropped out of school, he ended up homeless and then landed in jail for theft. Even though he was forced into a treatment program, he kept using drugs he managed to smuggle into jail, until one night he overdosed.

"I hallucinated and heard voices. I thought cell mates were talking to me when they really weren't—I tried to have 'conversations' with the voices I heard."

Stone said that for days he was out of touch with reality, trapped inside a frightening drug-induced world of his own. After that, even his cell mates told him he should quit. Eventually, he did quit, but it wasn't easy.

5

It's
Your Life

ric Stone got a second chance. At his sentencing hearing, four months after he went to jail, he was sentenced to an additional six months of jail time and required to successfully complete a treatment program after release.

Stone relapsed twice, but, he said, "I was sick of hurting all the time, and sick and tired of the addiction. I had experienced too much pain in my life, and doing drugs was no longer something that gave me pleasure—it was something that controlled my life."

Recovering from speed addiction isn't easy, Stone explained. Although it starts out as seemingly harmless and fun, it eventually takes over your life to the point where you can't imagine living without it—but you can't live with it either. Although recovery isn't easy, it isn't impossible either. People—such as Eric Stone— do get well.

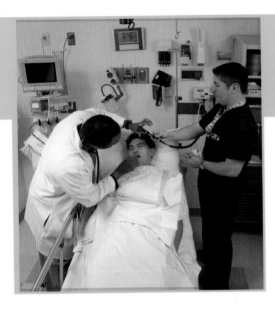

Speed users may have problems like malnutrition, tooth decay, and seizures, which must be treated before their addiction can be treated.

Treating Speed Addiction

Treating speed addicts poses special challenges. They've often been awake for days, so one of their first needs may be several nights of good sleep. During the first month after they've quit using speed, they may be more agitated and have a very short attention span. They also may suffer from psychiatric problems, like having delusions.

Many times they suffer from physical problems as well. They may have untreated wounds or advanced tooth decay, they can be malnourished, and they may suffer from seizures. Because of these special challenges, it can take speed addicts longer to recover than it might if they were addicted to some other substance.

The first goal of treatment is to stabilize the addict. Blood pressure and body temperature have to be checked. If either is too high, the user needs to be sent to a hospital. If the user is violent or out of control, he or she might have to be sedated.

Speed users often have other health problems that have to be dealt with. As noted earlier, they may have open sores that have become infected. They may have advanced tooth decay. They may be very thin and malnourished, or just generally run down.

After any immediate health concerns have been dealt with, the recovering user needs three essentials: sleep, lots of fluids, and healthy meals. Often a period of "planned sleep" is prescribed. The user might be allowed to sleep for four hours, then awakened and given fluids, then allowed to sleep for another four hours, and so on. Meals should include lots of fresh fruit, vegetables, and easily digestible protein such as eggs and yogurt.

The stabilization period during treatment can last for two to four weeks. During this time, users may experience paranoid thoughts and feelings. They may even become violent. To reduce the risk of violent outbursts, users are kept in a simple, quiet environment. Except when necessary, caregivers maintain a safe distance because closeness can be seen by the users as being threatening. For the same reason, they avoid jerky movements and keep their hands visible at all times. Conversations are conducted in low, calm voices. It's important to reassure the user that what he or she is feeling is a natural part of withdrawal.

Counseling Is Key

Once the addict is stable, counseling sessions can begin. In the early stages, the focus is on recovery skills: how to quit using speed, and how to avoid starting to use again. For instance, the counselor and patient will work together to identify the people, objects, and feelings in the patient's life that trigger speed use and figure out how to deal with those triggers.

Often these early sessions are short (because the patient may still be having trouble concentrating) but quite frequent (because the patient may also be having difficulty retaining what he or she has learned). Information is repeated to help the user remember what has been discussed.

Research has shown that the most successful treatments for speed involve the development of a positive relationship with a counselor, avoiding the company of other drug users, and becoming a member of a support group—a group of people who have similar experiences and can discuss ways to better cope with the treatment.

Effective treatment of speed addiction increases the patient's awareness of the effects of the drug; addresses his or her physical, psychological, and social problems; and involves family and friends. Treatment is usually more successful if the individual has the support of loved ones.

Hayley, whose story was mentioned previously, in chapter three, didn't exactly make her own choice to start treatment. Like Eric Stone, she was ordered into a treatment program after ending up in jail. She had to go to weekly counseling sessions and attend a day-treatment program. Her treatment program made her aware of the destructive pattern of drug use that she'd fallen into and helped her make some important changes in her life.

A vital part of that process was family counseling. "My parents and I had a lot of anger toward each other, and counseling has helped us to work

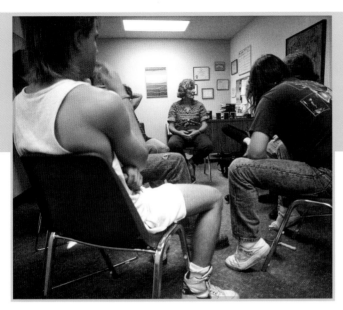

A counselor talks to young people in a support group. Counseling and therapy are vital to the successful treatment of speed addiction.

through that. We're starting to understand how we can relate to one another with more respect and tolerance, and we're learning to communicate without becoming hostile or freaking out," Hayley said.

Lisa's story of recovery also includes aspects of self-control. Lisa explained, "There've been a lot of ups and downs, but I haven't gone back to using. I am finally starting to feel my feelings instead of controlling them with drugs, and I'm finding other ways to cope with them."

People who use speed do get well, but it's a long, hard journey back to health from the frightening depths of addiction. As is true of all drug abuse, the best way to avoid the incredibly disgusting effects of addiction is never to misuse drugs at all. The more you learn about making the best and healthiest decisions in your life, the more you will be able to avoid those choices that bring you nothing but pain, suffering, and ruin.

Glossary

addiction Being abnormally tolerant to and dependent on something that is psychologically or physically habit-forming.

amphetamine A drug that is a stimulant and that was first manufactured in the nineteenth century.

antidepressant A medication that is used to treat depression, which is an overall feeling of sadness and hopelessness.

Benzedrine A form of ephedrine that once was sold without a prescription to treat nasal and bronchial congestion and was often used in inhalers; the first form of amphetamine to be abused.

dopamine A brain chemical that creates a feeling of pleasure.

ephedrine A stimulant derived from a shrub; the active substance in various Chinese traditional medicines.

formication The delusion that insects are crawling all over your skin.

hallucinations Imaginary visions and sounds.

methamphetamine A potent amphetamine that can be made into a powder or crystals. It causes the brain to release enormous amounts of dopamine.

meth mouth Nickname for the severe dental problems (including serious tooth decay) often associated with methamphetamine abuse.

neurons The nerve cells in the brain, made up of the cell body (which contains the nucleus), dendrites (which receive messages from other neurons), and axons (which pass messages to other neurons).

neurotransmitters Brain chemicals that pass signals from one neuron's axons to another neuron's dendrites.

paranoia A mental condition in which a person believes that someone or something is trying to harm him or her.

psychotic Relating to psychosis, a mental condition in which the sufferer loses touch with reality.

recovery skills The skills an addict needs in order to quit using and avoid starting using again.

relapse The use of drugs again after an attempt to give them up.

stimulant A substance that promotes wakefulness and alertness.

withdrawal The frequently unpleasant, and sometimes deadly, physical symptoms that a drug addict experiences after he or she stops using the drug.

For More Information

American Council for Drug Education
164 West 74th Street
New York, NY 10023
(800) 488-3784
Web site: http://www.acde.org
This organization offers educational programs and services to engage teens, address the needs of parents, and provide people with authoritative information on tobacco, alcohol, and drugs.

Canadian Centre on Substance Abuse (CCSA)
75 Albert Street, Suite 300
Ottawa, ON K1P 5E7
Canada
(613) 235-4048
Web site: http://www.ccsa.ca
The CCSA gathers and shares information on alcohol and other drug issues.

National Institute on Drug Abuse
National Institutes of Health
6001 Executive Boulevard, Room 5213
Bethesda, MD 20892-9561
(301) 443-1124

Web site: http://www.nida.nih.gov
NIDA, the U.S. government's focal point for research on drug abuse and addiction, aims to detect and respond to emerging drug abuse trends, understand how drugs work in the brain and body, and develop and test new treatment and prevention approaches.

Partnership for a Drug-Free America
405 Lexington Avenue, Suite 1601
New York, NY 10174
(212) 922-1560
Web site: http://www.drugfree.org
The Partnership for a Drug-Free America's mission is to reduce illicit drug use in America.

Web Sites

Due to the changing nature of Internet links, Rosen Publishing has developed an online list of Web sites related to the subject of this book. This site is updated regularly. Please use this link to access the list:

http://www.rosenlinks.com/idd/spee

For Further Reading

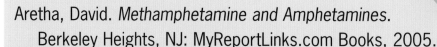

Aretha, David. *Methamphetamine and Amphetamines*. Berkeley Heights, NJ: MyReportLinks.com Books, 2005.

Berne, Emma Carlson. *Methamphetamine*. San Diego, CA: Reference Point Press, 2007.

Brady, Betty. *Meth Survivor: Jennifer's Story*. Bloomington, IN: Authorhouse, 2006.

Grabish, Beatrice R. *Drugs and Your Brain*. Center City, MN: Hazelden Publishing, 1998.

Harrow, Jeremy. *Crystal Meth* (Incredibly Disgusting Drugs). New York, NY: The Rosen Publishing Group, Inc., 2008.

Landau, Elaine. *Meth: America's Drug Epidemic*. Minneapolis, MN: Twenty-First Century Books, 2007.

Littell, Mary Ann. *Speed and Methamphetamine Drug Dangers*. Berkeley Heights, NJ: Enslow Publishers, 2000.

Marcovitz, Hal. *Drug Education Library—Methamphetamines*. Farmington Hills, MI: Lucent Books, 2005.

Mintzner, Richard. *Meth & Speed = Busted!* Berkeley Heights, NJ: Enslow Publishers, 2005.

Spalding, Frank. *Methamphetamine: The Dangers of Crystal Meth*. New York, NY: The Rosen Publishing Group, 2007.

Bibliography

Alberta Alcohol and Drug Abuse Commission. "ABCs of
  Amphetamines." Retrieved May 30, 2007 (http://www.
  aadac.com/documents/abcs_amphetamines.pdf).

Alberta Alcohol and Drug Abuse Commission. "Amphetamines:
  Beyond the ABCs." Retrieved May 30, 2007 (http://www.
  aadac.com/documents/beyond_abcs_amphetamines.pdf).

Alberta Alcohol and Drug Abuse Commission. "Crystal Meth and
  Youth: Effective Treatment and Prevention Practices."
  Retrieved May 30, 2007 (http://www.aadac.com/documents/
  crystal_meth_and_youth.pdf).

Aretha, David. *Methamphetamine and Amphetamines.* Berkeley
  Heights, NJ: MyReportLinks.com Books, 2005.

"Crystallized." *Drugs & Addiction Magazine*, Vol. D, Issue 1,
  pp. 31–39.

Deguire, Anne-Elyse. "Fact Sheet: Methamphetamine." Canadian
  Centre on Substance Abuse. 2005. Retrieved August 28,
  2007 (http://www.ccsa.ca/NR/rdonlyres/A378E355-BB39-
  45FB-BDB8-FB751EDBAFFD/0/ccsa0111342005.pdf).

Grabish, Beatrice R. *Drugs and Your Brain.* Center City, MN:
  Hazelden Publishing, 1998.

National Center for Drug-Free Sport. "Drugs in Sports:
  Amphetamines." Retrieved July 12, 2007 (http://www.
  drugfreesport.com/choices/drugs/amphetamine.html).

National Institute on Drug Abuse. "InfoFacts: Methamphetamine." Retrieved May 30, 2007 (http://www.drugabuse.gov/infofacts/ methamphetamine.html).

National Institute on Drug Abuse. "Mind Over Matter: Methamphetamine." Retrieved May 30, 2007 (http://teens.drugabuse.gov/mom/mom_ meth1.asp).

National Institute on Drug Abuse. "Research Report Series: Methamphetamine Abuse and Addiction." Retrieved May 30, 2007 (http://www.drugabuse.gov/ResearchReports/methamph/ methamph.html).

Naval Air Engineering Station Lakehurst. "Amphetamines." Retrieved July 12, 2007 (http://www.lakehurst.navy.mil/hro-lakehurst/dfwp/ amphetamines.htm).

Neuroscience for Kids. "Amphetamines." Retrieved July 12, 2007 (http:// faculty.washington.edu/chudler/amp.html).

Partnership for a Drug-Free America. Meth Information and Resource Centre. Retrieved August 28, 2007 (http://www.drugfree.org/Portal/ DrugIssue/MethResources/default.html).

Stone, Eric. "The Meth Trap." Partnership for a Drug-Free America. Retrieved May 30, 2007 (http://www.drugfree.org/Portal/DrugIssue/ MethResources/eric_stone.html).

Index

About the Author

Edward Willett lives in Regina, Saskatchewan, Canada. Among the books he has written are biographies of two famous rock stars, Jimi Hendrix and Janis Joplin, both of whom died at an early age as a result of drug abuse. Willett hopes that by contributing to the Incredibly Disgusting Drugs series, he can help prevent future drug-related tragedies.

Photo Credits

Cover, p. 1 © www.istockphoto.com/Joe Augustine; pp. 3, 10, 16, 22, 25, 27, 28, 32, 40, 42, 44, 45, 47 DEA; p. 7 © www.istockphoto.com/Cornel Krämer; p. 9 © Roger Viollet/ Getty Images; p. 13 © CNRI/Photo Researchers; p. 14 © Kairos, Latin Stock/ Photo Researchers; p. 17 © www.istockphoto.com/Jaun Estey; p. 18 American Dental Association; p. 21 © www.istockphoto.com/Marcel Pelletier; p. 23 © 2005 Faces of Meth; p. 29 © Scott Houston/Corbis; p. 31 © Getty Images; p. 33 National Library of Medicine/NIH; p. 36 © Spencer Grant/Photo Edit; p. 39 © Lawrence Migdale/Photo Researchers.

Designer: Les Kanturek; **Editor:** Kathy Kuhtz Campbell
Photo Researcher: Marty Levick